YOUR KNOWLEDGE HAS VALUE

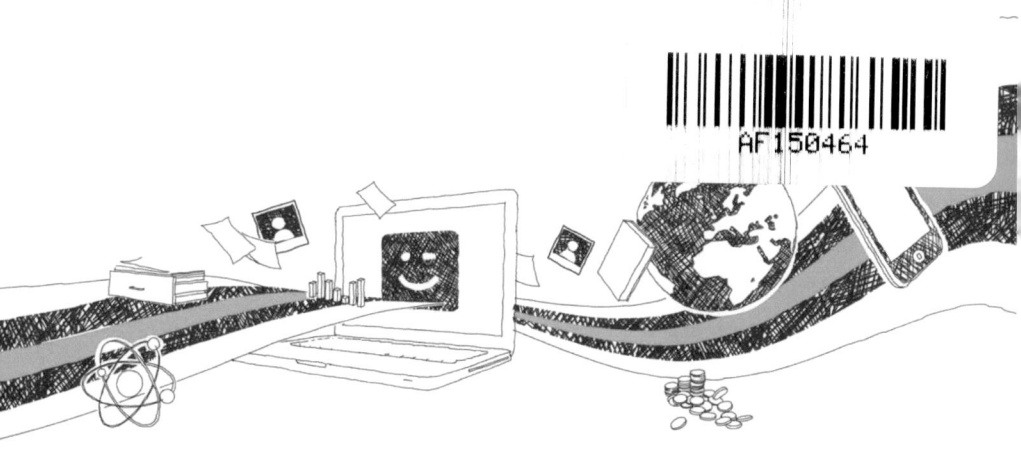

- We will publish your bachelor's and master's thesis, essays and papers

- Your own eBook and book - sold worldwide in all relevant shops

- Earn money with each sale

Upload your text at www.GRIN.com
and publish for free

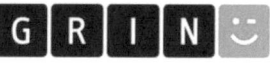

Bibliographic information published by the German National Library:

The German National Library lists this publication in the National Bibliography; detailed bibliographic data are available on the Internet at http://dnb.dnb.de .

Imprint:

Copyright © 2014 GRIN Verlag, Open Publishing GmbH
Print and binding: Books on Demand GmbH, Norderstedt Germany
ISBN: 9783656836759

This book at GRIN:

http://www.grin.com/en/e-book/283205/treatment-protocol-for-post-operative-endophthalmitis

Zia Mazhry

Treatment protocol for post operative endophthalmitis

Intravitreal Injections

GRIN Publishing

Endophthalmitis is a devastating complication of ocular surgery and trauma, which may lead to total loss of vision and sometimes even the eyeball. Management of endophthalmitis presents one of the most challenging problems in ophthalmology. Two third of all cases of endophthalmitis occur after surgery. 90% are caused by bacteria and the remaining 10% by fungi, viruses and parasites. Incidence reported in literature is 0.1% to 0.4%. Though no study is available, incidence in our setup seems to be even higher.

Traditionally endophthalmitis had been treated with topical and systemic antibiotics given both orally as well as parenterally but with poor therapeutic response. Another mode of treatment that has now become the standard treatment for endophthalmitis in developed countries is intravitreal injection of antimicrobials. Studies have proven this to be an effective, probably the only effective treatment available so far. In Pakistan this way treatment has not yet been widely practiced.

The authors have carried out a study on 56 eyes diagnosed as cases of endophthalmitis. The patients were treated with intravitreal injections. Results were encouraging. Anatomical integrity was preserved in 90% of cases and 60% had a visual acuity of 6/60 or better. A gold medal winning paper was presented by one of the authors in Ophthalmo 96 based on the above study. Great enthusiasm was shown about the technique. The Chairman of the conference advised to publish the technique.

The aim of this booklet is to present in a simple way the management of endophthalmitis using the technique of intravitreal injections. Secondly we want to decrease the undue hesitancy and fear about the use of intravitreal injections. By the end of the booklet the reader will feel confident to practice the procedure on his own whenever and wherever needed.

Diagnosis and Management Plan
For Endophthalmitis

Early symptoms.
Slight to no pain.
Decrease in visual acuity, which may be the only symptom.
Important.
Patient should be clearly told that vision is going to improve day by day and any deterioration after initial improvement must be taken seriously and immediately reported to the surgeon.
Late symptoms.
Severe pain.
Marked visual loss.
Lid edema.

Early signs.
Patient may present with minimal signs. Anterior chamber may be clear. Cells in vitreous may be the only finding on examination. This finding alone is sufficient to diagnose endophthalmitis in appropriate setting. One must have a routine look into the vitreous during postoperative examination since as already mentioned the patient may be absolutely symptom free.

Late signs.
Lid edema.
Chemosis.
Corneal haze.
Hypopyon.
Cells in the vitreous.
Absent red reflex.

Important.
The recognition of early symptoms and signs is the most important in the treatment of endophthalmitis. Late symptoms and signs do not mean that we should wait till the condition is established. Neither it means that the condition has become untreatable.

Management plan.

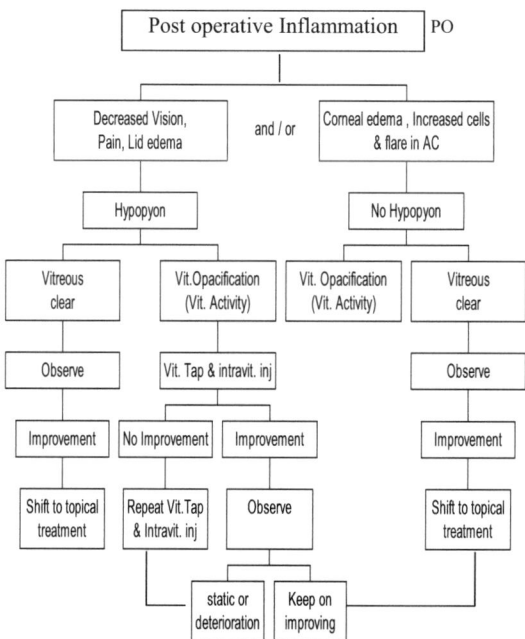

Doses and Preparation of Intravitreal Injections.

Antibacterials.

Drug	Dose	Spectrum
Amikacin	200-400 µg	Mainly G-ve.
Ampicillin	5 mg	Broad spectrum, mainly G +ve.
Carbenicillin	2 mg	G-ve.. Especially against Pseudomonas.
Cefazolin	2.25 mg	Broad spectrum, mainly G+ve.
Ceftazidime	2 mg	Mainly G-ve. Especially against Pseudomonas.
Gentamycin	200 µg	Mainly G-ve.
Kenamycin	300-500 µg	Mainly G-ve.
Lincomycin	1.50 mg	Mainly G +ve.
Oxacillin	0.5 mg	Resistant Staph.
Tobramycin	200-400 µg	Broad spectrum, mainly G-ve.
Vancomycin	1 mg	Resistant Staph.

3

Antifungals.

Drug	Dose
Amphotericin B	2-4 µg
Fluconazole	50 µg

Steroids.

Drug	Dose
Dexamethasone	200-400 µg

Preparation of intravitreal injections.

Generic name	Trade name	Original strength	Amount taken	Saline added	To make	Volume to be used
Cefazoline	Cefamezin Kefzol	250mg/5ml	0.2cc=10mg	0.3cc	0.5cc	0.1cc=2 mg
Ceftazidime	Fortum	500mg/5ml	0.1cc=10mg	0.4cc	0.5cc	0.1cc=2mg
Dexamethasone		4mg/ml	0.1cc=0.4mg			0.1cc=400µg
Fluconazole	Diflucan	2mg/ml	0.1cc=200µg	0.3cc	0.4cc	0.1cc=50µg
Gentamycin	Gentamycin	20mg/ml	0.1cc=200µg	0.9cc	1.0cc	0.1cc=200µg
Tobramycin	Nebcin	20mg/ml	0.1cc=200µg	0.9cc	1.0cc	0.1cc=200µg

- Injections should be prepared just before use. Left over quantity can be used to make fortified eye drops.
- Distilled water is required for the constitution of vials. BSS/Ringer's Lactate/Saline is used for dilutions
- Expiry for the constituted vial is one week or as specified by the manufacturer if distilled water is used.
- Discard the dilutions after single use.

Procedure and Technique.

Choice of antimicrobials

Time of onset gives some clue to the type of organism.
- Staph aureus and gram-negative organisms usually present between first and third postoperative days with severe signs.
- Staph. Epidermidis usually presents with mild signs between fourth and tenth postoperative days.
- Fungus generally presents around third post op. week with mild signs.

When no stain or culture or gram stain report is available an antibiotic combination which covers both gram positive and gram negative organisms along with a steroid is used.

For Example.
Cefazolin+Tobramycin+Dexamethasone
OR
Vancomycin+Ceftazidime+Dexamethasone
OR
Vancomycin+Cefazolin+Tobramycin+Ceftazidime
+Dexamethasone

Steroid is used in a routine cover but must not to be used if a fungal infection is suspected.
All the antifungal drugs are very toxic and should not be used until there is a very strong suspicion or positive staining or culture report for the fungus.

Anesthesia.
- Choice of anesthesia depends on the surgeon and the patient. Intravitreal injection can be given under topical anesthesia. Another method is to give the anesthetic agent subconjunctivally at the site of injection.
- If the patient is apprehensive or feels excessive pain surgeon should not hesitate to give retrobulbar or peribulbar anesthesia.

Site.
Injection site is 3.5mm posterior to the limbus in aphakic and 4.0mm posterior to the limbus in phakic eyes.

Vitreous aspiration and injection
To give the injection we use a 1cc syringe with detachable needle of size between 24G to 27G.The bigger gauge needle is required in younger patients and in cases where the vitreous abscess is thicker and difficult to aspirate. Tip of the needle is directed towards the centre of the vitreous cavity. First the vitreous is aspirated. If vitreous cannot be aspirated AC tap should be performed. Never try to inject without aspiration. After aspiration the syringe is removed holding the needle in place with an artery forceps. Now the syringe containing the antibiotic is attached to the same needle and injected. All the steps are performed under sterile conditions using sterile ingredients and aseptic technique. Volume of each injection is 0.05 to 0.1cc.with total injectable volume in the range of 0.1 to 0.3cc.

In cases where vitreous aspiration is not possible and we have to resort to AC tap, the final injectable volume should be kept as little as possible. This can be done by making each injection in a volume of 0.05cc instead of 0.1cc. To achieve this, the same guidelines should be followed as already given in the table.

Precautions.
- Great care should be taken while preparing the injections. Low dose will result in inadequate response whereas higher doses are toxic for the retina.
- Sterility should be maintained throughout.
- Injection site should be accurately determined using a caliper. Too anterior injection may result in hemorrhage. Too posterior injection may lead to retinal detachment.
- Tip of the needle should be pointed towards the centre of the vitreous cavity.
- Tip of the needle should not be more than 1 to 1.25cm in the vitreous cavity.
- Do not inject if you are unable to aspirate the vitreous. Instead go for an AC tap and inject into the vitreous.
- Inject slowly and steadily. Injection jet may damage the retina.

Follow up.

After intravitreal injection, the patient should be examined everyday. Points that require special consideration include vitreous activity, degree of hypopyon, and fundal glow. Increasing or static vitreous activity indicates insufficient treatment. Injection should be repeated after 24 hours without hesitation if response is not adequate. Up to 6 injections have been given in one of our cases with successful outcome.

Prognostic signs.
Good prognostic signs.
- Decreasing activity in vitreous.
- Decreasing hypopyon.
- Clearing anterior chamber.
- Decreasing corneal edema.
- Improving fundal glow

Important.

If vitreous activity or haze is increasing one should never be deceived by clear anterior chamber or other signs.

Poor prognostic signs.
- Increasing vitreous activity or opacification.
- Increasing hypopyon.
- Increasing cells and flare in AC.
- Increasing corneal edema.
- Absent fundal glow.

If the condition is static or is deteriorating repeat intravitreal injection. If the condition is improving shift to topical treatment.

Role of vitreous lavage.

Vitreous lavage is an ideal substitute for vitrectomy. It can be undertaken in cases where vitreous is easy to aspirate i.e. in fluid vitreous as in old age and when the patient is already vitrectomised.

Procedure.

Two 10cc syringes are used with 24G to 26G needles. BSS taken in one syringe is injected and the fluid aspirated through the other at the same time. Site is same as in intravitreal injection with the exception that instead of one, two sites opposite to each other are used. At the end of the procedure intravitreal injection is given in a similar way as described above.

Role of Pars Plana Vitrectomy.

- The recommendation of Endophthalmitis Vitrectomy Study group is to do an immediate vitrectomy if the visual acuity is reduced to perception of light only.
- Our experience, however, is to do a vitrectomy if we are not able to aspirate the vitreous with a 23G needle assuming that the vitreous abscess is too thick to be aspirated. By vitrectomy we mean a core vitrectomy and the case should be referred to an expert posterior segment surgeon.

Complications of therapy.

Inadequacies

Improper technique may result in complications as already mentioned in precautions. Rate of complications approaches to almost nil if proper care is exercised. Especially important is that an injection should not be given if vitreous cannot be aspirated.

Retinal and Macular Toxicity

Infectious process itself and the treatment available both are toxic for the retina and the macula but when the question is to save the eye these factors should not be excessive weight. Anything less than evisceration and phthisical eye should be considered an achievement. Many eyes have been saved using multiple injections and a post treatment vision of 6/6.

Others

Definitely we loose some eyes due to iatrogenic retinal detachment, perforation but mainly due to uncontrolled infection. Nothing can be said precisely about the cause in each case.

Outcome

In our study we could achieve 6/6 to 6/24 vision in 30%of cases. 26% had 6/36 to 6/60. Anatomical integrity could be preserved in more than 90%.

Considering the pros and cons and risk benefit ratio, intravitreal injections and pars plana vitrectomy remains the only choice by which we can hope some good results.

In the end we want to mention the conclusion of the EVS that antibiotics presently available if given systemically will only lead to increased toxic effects, costs and hospital stay, so they should better be avoided.

Conclusions.

- One should have a high index of suspicion for endophthalmitis while examining the patients post operatively.

- If one is unable to differentiate between bacterial and sterile endophthalmitis, the condition must be treated as bacterial endophthalmitis.

- Whenever endophthalmitis is suspected, immediate vitreous aspiration combined with intravitreal injection of antibiotics and steroids is recommended.

- The corner stone of clinical diagnosis is VITREOUS activity and opacification and the corner stone of treatment is optimum concentration of antibiotics inside the battle field i.e. the VITREOUS.

Further reading.

1. Pravan PR: Shotgun therapy for exogenous endophthalmitis, University of South Florida. Tampa. USA. 1-2, 1997.
2. Slamovit T.L: American Academy of Ophthalmology, Basic and Clinical Science Course Section 9, Intraocular Inflammation and Uveitis, 141-144, San Francisco, 1995-96.
3. Kanski JJ, editor: Clinical Ophthalmology. A Systematic Approach, 300-302, Oxford, 1994. Butterworth Heinemann.
4. Krupin T, Kolker AE, editors: Atlas of Complications of Ophthalmic Surgery, London, 1993, The CV Mosby Co.
5. Berger BB, The Lens, Cataract and its Management, Peymann GA, Sanders DR, Goldberg MF, editors, Principles and Practice of Ophthalmology, Vol. 1, 599-601, Philadelphia, 1980, W.B. Saunders Company.

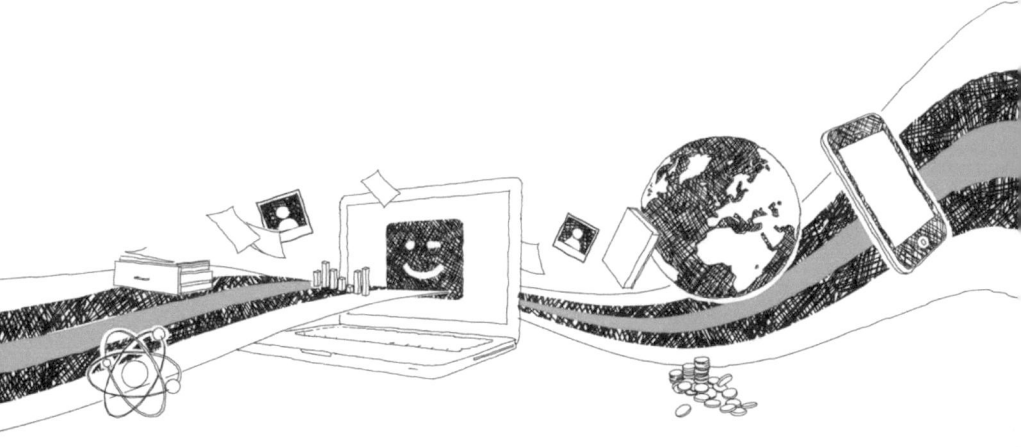
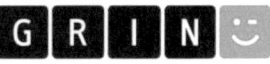